21-DAY EFFECTIVE COLITIS AND CRO1

An anti inflammatory diet guide and cookbook with over 150 plant-based, belly-soothing recipes to help heal inflammatory bowel disease.

Table of Contents

INTRODUCTION

Ulcerative colitis: Even the name is scary. But let's break it down. UC is a chronic autoimmune infection that causes inflammation of the colon (part of colitis) and rectum. This inflammation can cause an ulcer (the part of the UC) on the intestinal wall or open sores, which can lead to bleeding and leakage of pus and mucus. Resulting to symptoms, such as severe and frequent diarrhea and pain. You may hear the term "colitis", but you should know that ulcerative colitis and "colitis" are completely different. Colitis is a short-term inflammation of the colon, while ulcerative colitis is a more serious chronic disease.

UC has the same effect on men and women UC is one of the two main types of inflammatory bowel disease (IBD). Crohn's disease is another. Although Crohn's and UC are similar, there are some key differences. The main difference is that UC is usually associated with concentrated inflammation in the large intestine, while Crohn's bacteria may affect any part of the digestive tract.

Common Symptoms

These signs are complications, which are not directly caused by the inflammation in the colon. These complications are general symptoms and signs of soreness and they include;

- Weakness

- Arthritis

- Fever

- Bloody stool

- Nausea

- Skin sores

Risk factors for ulcerative colitis include:

- **Genetics**: UC often arises in families, however according to an article in "The Lancet", a number of genetic differences have been identified in people with IBD. If you have a parent or a sibling with a disease, your own risk will be increased 10-fold. But even with that big jump, it's still hardly that you're going to develop it: only about 10% to 25% of people with UC have a first-degree IBD relative (either UC or Crohn's).

- **Age:** UC normally begins first in people between the ages of 15 and 30. It is also more likely to develop in individuals over 60 years of age, possibly due to the aging of the immune system and the body as a whole.

- **Race and ethnicity**: UC tend to affect people of all races and ethnicities, the Caucasian and Ashkenazi people of Jewish descent are at higher risk.

LIFESTYLE CHANGES THAT CAN HELP

You can also find relief by creating changes to your daily life, including physical activity, diet, and more. Here are some areas that need to be focused on:

- **Exercise**: Research shows that physical activity can be of great help to people with UC, helping to boost the immune system, promote healing, and reduce stress.

- **Sleep**: Getting quality night's sleep is important for people with UC who may already be struggling with fatigue due to iron deficiency and other side effects. If you're battling to get enough rest, getting your digestive symptoms under control can help.

- **Diet**. There is no exact "UC diet". You may discover that some foods trigger your UC symptoms more than others. Common ones include high-fat foods, sugary foods, and insoluble fiber foods. Keeping a food diary can enable you figure it out. Consult your doctor or registered dietitian to figure out a meal plan that works for you.

- **Mental health**: Living with a serious disease like UC raises your risk of mental health problems, such as depression and anxiety. You may need to consider seeing a therapist to help guide you through the stress of UC.

ULCERATIVE COLITIS AND DIET

UC can reduce your appetite. In this article, We will help you understand the role food plays in symptoms and how to ensure that food helps you heal and not hurt.

Supplements for UC

When you have a disease like UC, it seems to turn your digestive system into a hot nightmare, and food will feel like a jealous burning. Truly, diet does not cause ulcerative colitis, which affects the colon and rectum, but certain foods may trigger symptoms of UC. Knowing exactly how nutrition and diet affect UC management can be tricky, but read on to learn about things to avoid and things to continue to enjoy.

Diet and Nutrition

We consulted some of the top UC experts in the United States to provide you with the most scientific and up-to-date information. In fact, there are no set of trigger food lists that apply to everyone with UC.

Just as everyone's UC symptoms are unique, so are their problem foods. So, what should you do? Find a guide that suits you.

The best way to figure out how to make a diet suitable for UC is to seek advice from a registered dietitian. Ask your gastroenterologist (GI) if they can recommend you to an R.D. they trust.

Diet cannot cure the inflammation completely, but it can significantly improve symptoms. For instance, a low FODMAPs diet can improve gas, bloating, and certain types of abdominal pain or irritation.

Common Foods to avoid with IBD

- **Lactose:** With age, many people lose the ability to digest lactose. Lactose is a sugar in dairy products. You may notice that when you consume it, your UC symptoms will also increase. Therefore, you may wish to limit your milk and cheese intake. If you prefer milk, please choose lactose-free milk. Otherwise, try almond or oat milk. Remember that Greek yogurt is low in lactose. It may be wise to incorporate it into your diet because of the probiotics it contains can be essential to your gut by helping maintain a healthy bacteria balance and it is good source of protein. Dairy is a -inflammatory trigger food and that is a good reason to avoid it.

  Sugary foods: Foods and beverages with high sugar content may increase the body's inflammatory response and change the balance of healthy bacteria in the abdomen, thereby worsening UC symptoms. Try to limit your intake of soda, juice, candies, pastries and other foods high in sweets. Besides, as you know, this is not best for your well-being.

- **Alcohol**: Based on a study by Alcohol Research. When you have UC, your gastrointestinal tract has been irritated, and alcohol will only cause more harm. In addition, many alcoholic beverages contain too much sugar, which makes the problem even more complicated. Avoiding alcohol, or drinking alcohol only on special occasions can help. Even so, women only drink one bottle a day, and men drink two glasses a day, instead of ordering a sugared cocktail and mixed drink, drink a glass of wine or beer.

- **Caffeine**: In some people with UC, the caffeine in coffee, soda, and other beverages can aggravate the inflamed bowel wall. In addition, it can speed up the entire digestive system and make your body unhealthier.

- **High-fat foods**: Super-fat foods can cause serious damage to some people's UC symptoms by increasing inflammation in the digestive tract. Pay attention to foods containing butter, butter, margarine and coconut, and limit the intake of fat, greasy and fried foods.

- **Insoluble fiber foods**: Some people with UC may find that foods containing insoluble fiber may be difficult to digest and cause symptoms such as diarrhea. These foods may include fruits with skins and seeds, whole nuts, whole grains, unprocessed green and cruciferous vegetables such as broccoli and cauliflower. Oftentimes, people say that they follow a "low residue diet" to reduce UC symptoms. Basically, this is another way of saying they restrict high-fiber foods. If you have been diagnosed with stenosis or recently had surgery, you should also avoid these foods.

- **Spicy food**: Abstain from hot sauce! You may also find that foods with "spicy" are not well placed in the digestive tract. It is because they contain capsaicin, capsaicin acts as a stimulant and legally heats the intestinal wall. Moreover, since UC has already caused damage to your colon, more stimulation from this kind hot spice is the last thing your body needs.

FODMAP Food

You may also have heard of something called a low FODMAP diet (here is the absurd full name: fermentable oligosaccharides, disaccharides, monosaccharides and polyols). FODMAPs are carbohydrates that are absorbed in the small intestine. When they land in the colon, colonic bacteria ferment undigested sugars to produce gas. Some studies have shown that following this diet can help reduce inflammation.

High FODMAP foods include:

- Lactose foods
- Rye, wheat and barley
- Foods with fructose like apples, honey, and pears
- Foods that contain polyols, like stone fruits, mushrooms and cauliflower

Low FODMAP foods include:

- Almond and soy milk
- Cantaloupe, grapes, kiwi
- Eggs, tofu, plain lean meats
- Cucumber, potato, zucchini

You may want to incorporate low FODMAP foods during the flare, but before you try, please contact your R.D. for advice before getting started.

Eating during a IBD Flare: Tips

Simply prepare food: Yes, this is simple code. Instead of frying food or immersing it in a lot of oil, choose steaming, grilling or boiling food.

Stay hydrate: For patients with IBD, hydration is particularly important, because all diarrhea may dehydrate IBD, and diarrhea consumes electrolytes in the body. Make sure to drink plenty of water throughout the day and choose general hydrating foods such as soups. A good way to tell you if there are enough fluids is to check the color of your urine; it should range from light yellow to clear. Darker yellow is a sign that you need to drink even more.

Choose low-fiber fruits: Although certain fruits (such as apples, oranges, and peaches) can hardly tolerate UC due to their insoluble fiber content, low-fiber foods such as cantaloupe, nectar, and bananas have a milder effect on the stomach. Cooking fruits can also make them easier to digest. Fruits made into smoothies can also be eaten.

Choose vegetables wisely: Vegetables are a key part of any diet, but when you have UC, you should pay attention to which vegetables to eat and how to eat them. Choose non-cruciferous vegetables (usually healthy choices, but they are notorious gas-producing plants, which are exactly what you don't want during the flare) and skinless and seedless choices such as asparagus tips, potatoes and squash. Fully cooked vegetables can also help you digest them more easily.

Go for refined grains: Foods such as white rice, white pasta, and oatmeal may be easier to digest during an outbreak. On the other hand, whole grains and whole nuts contain a lot of insoluble fiber, which can be difficult to digest.

Incorporate lean proteins: Poultry and other meats with thin slices of lean meat, as well as fish, soybeans, eggs, and tofu, can complement the UC diet well and help you get the protein your body needs. This is important, especially if you have been losing weight.

Stick to "safe" food: If you find a meal or two that you can successfully endure during an outbreak, keep that knowledge in your diary. (Hope you will know what it is, because you have been following it!) Sometimes, you already know some light meal and snack ideas that suit you can help.

Eating during Remission

Relief period; such a happy time, when you are not harassed internally, you may wonder if you can "relax" a little bit more about the food you eat. Generally, you should move slowly when adding new food to your diet during remission. In fact, it is best to do it once at a time so that you can monitor any reaction. Otherwise, strive to achieve the essentials of the Mediterranean diet (tolerable!) to get the nutrients you need. Your doctor or R.D. can also provide more advice. In the meantime:

- ✓ Limit intake of processed foods
- ✓ Incorporate poultry, fish, beans and eggs weekly
- ✓ Consume moderate portions of dairy if you can tolerate lactose
- ✓ Limit your consumption of red meat

✓ Prioritize whole grains, low-fiber fruits, non-cruciferous vegetables and healthy fats

UC and Nutritional Supplements

Your gastrointestinal or registered dietitian will recommend supplements based on your specific situation after reviewing the symptoms and test results. Before adding supplements to your daily care, be sure to ask your doctor for permission. Certain supplements may actually contain sugar alcohols, lactose, and preservatives, which can actually aggravate your symptoms.

Having said that, these are some supplements that are usually recommended for people with UC. Don't forget to eat first before taking them, otherwise they may irritate your gastrointestinal tract:

o **Iron**: People living with UC may end up losing a fair amount of blood through their stool due to bleeding ulcers in their colon, raising their risk of iron deficiency anemia. In fact, this is the most obvious complication of IBD and affects approximately 45 per cent of patients, according to a research in Therapeutic Advances in Gastroenterology. Having a low red blood cell count not only makes it more difficult for your cells to get the oxygen they deserve, but it actually leaves you feeling exhausted as well.

o **Methotrexate**: If you are consuming certain drugs for UC, including 5aminosalicylate-acid sulfasalazine, your body may have problems absorbing folic acid as a natural consequence. This is not ideal, as folic acid helps promote healthy cell growth in the body, among other important functions. If you are taking one of these medications, or if you are pregnant or plan to become pregnant, your doctor will probably recommend folic acid supplementation.

o **Vitamin D and calcium**: For all individuals with UC and IBD in general, vitamin D is prescribed because there is some evidence that it can help with inflammation in the bowels. In fact, one review in Clinical Gastroenterology and Hepatology revealed that being deficient in vitamin D may increase your risk of relapse during UC remission. This is a vitamin that can be difficult for anyone to get from food on their own. If you are low in vitamin D, your doctor may recommend that you take a supplement. Make sure you ask them how much you should take per day, and pair it with calcium to help support your bone health. Calcium is especially if you have steroids that can increase your risk of weakened bones (osteoporosis).

PLANT-BASED BELLY-SOOTHING RECIPES FOR IBD

BREAKFAST RECIPES

Whole-Grain Morning Glory Muffins

These healthy breakfast treats have walnuts, which may offer protection against ulcerative colitis. Walnuts contain omega-3 fatty acids, eating them will offer preventative benefits in UC patients, resulting less damage from inflammation leading up to flare, plus faster healing after. Take note of any recipes with

Serving Size: 12

Prep and Cook Time: 1 hr.

INGREDIENTS

- 3 large eggs
- ½ cup raisins
- 2 cups white whole-wheat flour
- 2 tsp. baking soda
- 2 tsp. ground cinnamon
- 1 tsp. ground cardamom
- 1 tsp. ground ginger
- Cooking spray
- ¼ tsp. kosher salt
- ¾ cup unsweetened applesauce
- ½ cup vegetable oil

- ½ cup pure maple syrup
- 2 tsp. vanilla extract
- ½ cup chopped walnuts
- 1 cup finely grated carrots

Nutrition Information

Per Serving: *260 Calories; 15g Fat; 2g Saturated Fat; 45mg Cholesterol;*
277mg Sodium; 30g Carbohydrate; 3g Fiber; 5g Protein; 14g Sugar; 37mg Calcium; 1mg Iron; 215mg Potassium

Directions

STEP 1

Preheat your oven to 350°F. Grease your 12 muffin cups, or arrange with paper liners.

STEP 2

In a sizeable bowl, combine together flour, baking soda, cinnamon, cardamom, ginger, and salt. Set aside.

STEP 3

In a separate bowl, whisk eggs, applesauce, oil, maple syrup, and vanilla until combined. Stir in carrots.

STEP 4

Pour wet ingredients into dry ingredients; stir until just well mixed. Fold in raisins and walnuts.

STEP 5

Divide the batter equally into your prepared muffin tins. Bake in preheated oven for 20 minutes, or until a toothpick inserted in the center of a muffin comes out mostly clean. Allow to cool for 15 minutes before removing from muffin tin and transfer to a wire rack to cool completely, and then serve. Store the remaining in an air-tight container or refrigerate

Peanut Butter-Banana Green Smoothie

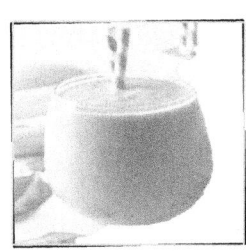 Consider using this low FODMAP milkshake for your all-in-one breakfast. Ulcerative colitis can destroy your ability to absorb nutrients. This smoothie can help you get the essentials you need: Spinach is a good source of iron-a mineral that is at risk of deficiency in UC flares. Banana helps to replace lost nutrients like potassium, which is important for electrolyte balance.

Serving Size 1

Prep and Cook Time: 5 min.

INGREDIENTS

- 1 cup fresh spinach

- 1 medium frozen banana, sliced
- ¼ cup old-fashioned rolled oats
- ½ tsp. ground cinnamon
- 1 cup unsweetened vanilla soymilk
- 1 Tbsp. natural salted peanut butter

Nutrition Information

Per Serving: *385 Calories; 14g Fat; 2g Saturated Fat; 0mg Cholesterol;*
182mg Sodium; 51g Carbohydrate; 9g Fiber; 16g Protein; 16g Sugar; 377mg Calcium; 4mg Iron; 801mg Potassium

DIRECTION

STEP 1

Mix all the ingredients in a high powder blender; blend until smooth. Served topped with strawberries (if desired).

Avocado-Egg Salad Toast

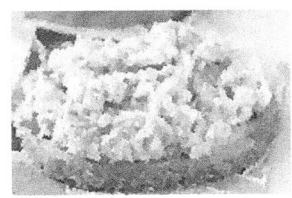 Give your eggs an extra dose to fight omega-3s. Avocados can help replenish the potassium lost due to diarrhea caused by UC flares. This is when you really want to choose whole wheat bread

instead of white bread: it has a lower fiber content and is easier
to digest

Serving Size: 4

Prep and Cook Time: 10 min.

INGREDIENTS

- 1 large ripe avocado
- ¼ tsp. black pepper
- 4 hard-boiled eggs, diced
- 1 Tbsp. fresh lemon juice
- ½ tsp. kosher salt
- 4 slices white sourdough bread, toasted
- 1 Tbsp. chopped fresh parsley, plus more for garnish

Nutrition Information

Per serving: *328 Calories; 14g Fat; 3g Saturated Fat; 186mg Cholesterol; 700mg Sodium; 38g Carbohydrate; 5g Fiber; 14g Protein; 4g Sugar; 66mg Calcium; 4mg Iron; 397mg Potassium*

DIRECTIONS

STEP 1

Cut the avocado in half and then remove the core. Remove the flesh from the skin and put it in a bowl. Mash thoroughly using a fork. Add the diced eggs, lemon juice, parsley, salt and pepper.

STEP 2

Divide mixture equally onto each slice of toasted bread. Garnish with additional parsley, if desired.

Fluffy Blueberry Oatmeal Pancakes

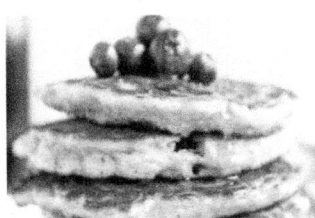

Whole wheat flour and oatmeal can provide a double dose of whole wheat food, which can enhance the body's anti-inflammatory compounds.

Serving Size: 3

Prep and Cook Time: 30 min.

INGREDIENTS

- ½ cup quick-cooking oats
- ¾ cup white whole-wheat flour
- 1 tsp. baking powder
- Cooking spray
- ½ tsp. ground cinnamon
- ¼ tsp. salt

- 1 large egg, whisked
- 4 Tbsp. pure maple syrup, divided
- 1 Tbsp. vegetable oil
- ½ tsp. vanilla extract
- 2 Tbsp. creamy almond butter
- ¾ cup unsweetened cashew milk (or your non-dairy milk of choice) ⬚½ cup frozen wild blueberries, thawed, plus more for garnish

Nutrition Information

Per serving: *389 Calories; 15g Fat; 2g Saturated Fat; 62mg Cholesterol; 453mg Sodium; 54g Carbohydrate; 7g Fiber; 10g Protein; 18g Sugar; 166mg Calcium; 3mg Iron; 226mg Potassium*

DIRECTIONS

STEP 1

Mix the oats and cashew milk in a medium bowl; allow for few minutes to coat.

STEP 2

Afterwards, combine flour, baking powder, cinnamon, and salt in a large bowl; stir with a whisk. Keep aside.

STEP 3

Add 1 Tbsp. of the maple syrup, oil, egg and vanilla to oat mixture; stir to mix well. Pour in the oat mixture into flour mixture; stir until just well mixed. Fold in blueberries.

STEP 4

Heat a greased nonstick skillet or griddle over medium heat. As the pan heats, mix the remaining 3 Tbsp. maple syrup and almond butter in a small bowl. Add 1 Tbsp. hot water and stir using a whisk until smooth. Keep aside.

STEP 5

Place a scant ¼ cup of pancake batter per pancake onto hot griddle. Bake until tops are covered with bubbles and edges look dry and cooked, about 3 minutes. Flip and cook 1 to 2 minutes on the other side.

STEP 6

Serve with almond butter sauce and additional blueberries, if needed.

Southwestern Sweet Potato and Egg Hash

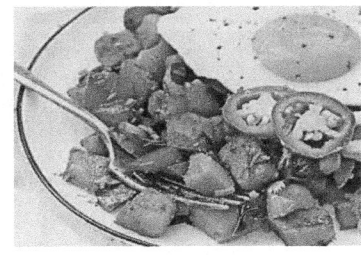

This antioxidant-rich breakfast will start the day! Breakfast hash is a great way to increase vegetable intake, which is one of the pillars of the Mediterranean diet. This is a

23

double vitamin A that combines sweet potato and red bell pepper, which
many UC patients lack.

Serving Size: 2

Prep and Cook Time: 25 min.

INGREDIENTS

- 2 large eggs
- 2 ½ Tbsp. extra-virgin olive oil, divided
- ¾ cup chopped red bell pepper
- ¼ tsp. ground cumin
- ¼ cup finely chopped red onion
- ½ tsp. chili powder
- ½ tsp. kosher salt, divided
- 4 Tbsp. prepared salsa
- ½ ripe avocado, well sliced
- Fresh cilantro for garnish (optional)
- 2 cups peeled and cubed sweet potato (about ½-in. each)

Nutrition Information

Per serving: *458 Calories; 29g Fat; 5g Saturated Fat; 185mg Cholesterol; 746mg Sodium; 35g Carbohydrate; 9g Fiber; 10g Protein; 10g Sugar; 84mg Calcium; 2mg Iron; 960mg Potassium*

DIRECTIONS

STEP 1

Heat 1 Tbsp. oil in a large skillet over medium. Add sweet potato; cook for 5 minutes, until lightly golden. Add 3 Tbsp. water, cover, and cook until tender, stirring occasionally for about 7 minutes.

STEP 2

Add 1 Tbsp. oil, onion and bell pepper to pan with potatoes. Cook uncovered, for about 5 minutes until vegetables are tender. Season with ¼ tsp. of the salt, chili powder and cumin; divide mixture between two bowls.

STEP 3

Add remaining ½ tsp. oil to pan. Crack eggs into pan; cook for 3 to 4 minutes, or until whites are set. Season with remaining ¼ tsp. salt.

STEP 4

Place an egg on top of each potato mixture. Top each with 2 Tbsp. salsa, sliced avocado, and cilantro for garnish. Serve.

Orange-Scented Golden Overnight Oats

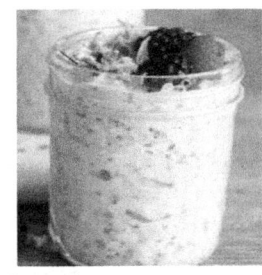

Put these oats in the refrigerator before going to bed and wake up to a delicious breakfast! The color of this dish comes from turmeric, which contains anti-inflammatory compounds, which may be beneficial for the treatment of ulcerative colitis. To get a double anti-inflammatory effect, add some berries, such as raspberries or
blueberries, to the oatmeal.

Serving Size: 2

Prep and Cook Time: 6 hr. 5 min.

INGREDIENTS

- 2 Tbsp. pure maple syrup
- 1 cup old-fashioned rolled oats
- 1 ¼ cup unsweetened vanilla soymilk
- 1 tsp. orange zest
- ¼ tsp. kosher salt
- ¾ tsp. ground turmeric
- ¼ tsp. ground cinnamon

Optional topping

- Fresh raspberries and/or blueberries

Nutrition Information

Per serving: *261 Calories; 6g Fat; 1g Saturated Fat; 0mg Cholesterol; 296mg Sodium; 43g Carbohydrate; 6g Fiber; 9g Protein; 14g Sugar; 241mg Calcium; 3mg Iron; 373mg Potassium*

DIRECTIONS

STEP 1

Combine the all ingredients (except the berries if using) in a container or Mason jar; stir well. Cover and refrigerate for 6 hours, or overnight. Garnish with fresh berries, if needed.

Smoked-Salmon Breakfast Bake

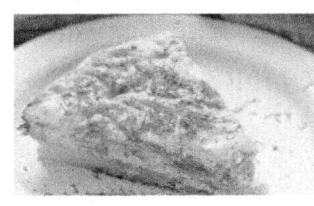

Salmon and eggs are good sources of vitamin D for bone strengthening, and many people with UC lack vitamin D. Studiesprove that this fat-soluble vitamin can also help relieve Inflammation of the guts.

Serving Size: 6

Prep and Cook Time: 50 min.

INGREDIENTS

- ¼ tsp. salt
- 10 large eggs
- 1 tsp. Dijon mustard
- ¼ tsp. black pepper
- 2 Tbsp. extra-virgin olive oil
- 2 oz. goat cheese, well crumbled
- ¼ cup finely chopped red onion
- 2 Tbsp. minced fresh chives, divided
- 12 oz. russet potatoes, peeled and cut into ½ in. cubes
- 6 oz. hot-smoked salmon, flaked (find it near the fresh-fish counter) **Nutrition Information**

Per serving: *295 Calories; 18g Fat; 6g Saturated Fat; 338mg Cholesterol;*
518mg Sodium; 12g Carbohydrate; 1g Fiber; 21g Protein; 1g Sugar; 85mg Calcium; 2mg Iron; 505mg Potassium

DIRECTIONS

STEP 1

Preheat oven to 350°F.

STEP 2

Put 1 Tbsp. chives, eggs, mustard, salt, and pepper in a sizable bowl; whisk to well combine. Keep aside.

STEP 3

Heat oil in a 10-inch oven-safe skillet over medium temperature. Add the potatoes, stir well to coat, arrange in a single layer. Cover and cook until potatoes are almost done, about 8 minutes, stirring occasionally. Add red onion; cook for additional 3 minutes, until softened.

STEP 4

Place the salmon equally over potato mixture in pan. Pour egg mixture over salmon and potatoes. Drizzle cheese on top, and place pan to preheated oven. Bake until egg for 25 minutes, or until mixture is set.

STEP 6

Garnish with remaining 1 Tbsp. chives. Allow to cool for 5 minutes before cutting into 6 slices. Serve.

Spinach and Red-Pepper Muffin-Tin Frittatas

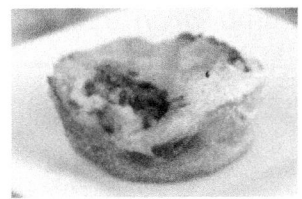

Eggs are an important source of protein and are usually well tolerated during attacks of ulcerative colitis. For extra anti-inflammatory ability, choose a brand that has fortified omega-3 fatty acids. Eat a batch of these low FODMAP eggs throughout the week.

Serving Size: 6

Prep and Cook Time: 40 min.

INGREDIENTS

- 12 large eggs
- Cooking spray
- 1 tsp. kosher salt
- 4 oz. fresh spinach
- 2 tsp. olive oil
- ½ tsp. black pepper
- frozen shredded hash browns
- 1 red bell pepper, well chopped
- Fresh avocado slices for serving (optional)
- 12 oz. refrigerated unseasoned shredded hash brown potatoes (or use thawed

Nutrition Information

Per serving: *217 calories; 11g fat; 3g saturated fat; 372mg cholesterol; 514mg sodium; 14g carbohydrate; 2g fiber; 15g protein; 1g sugar; 75mg calcium; 2mg iron; 272mg potassium*

DIRECTIONS

STEP 1

Preheat your oven to 400°F. Divide potatoes equally into 12 greased muffin cups; press into bottoms and slightly up sides. Bake for 15 minutes, or until lightly golden.

STEP 2

Afterwards, heat oil in a sizeable skillet over medium temperature. Add bell pepper, and cook until softened, about 5 to 6 minutes. Add spinach, and cook until wilted, stirring frequently, about 1 minute. Spread the vegetable mixture equally in each muffin tin over cooked potatoes.

STEP 3

Whisk the eggs, add salt, and pepper in a large bowl, and pour equally into each muffin cup. Place back in the oven and heat until eggs are just set, about 10 to 12 minutes. Allow to cool for 5 minutes before removing from pan.

STEP 4

Serve with sliced avocado, if desired. Refrigerate leftovers in an air tight bag; reheat in a microwave or toaster oven.

LUNCH RECIPES

Tahini-Caesar Chicken Pitas

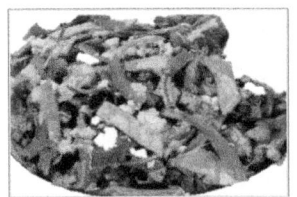 Since many UC patients suffer from dairy intolerance, this Caesar seasoning is made with tahini. Tahini is a sesame paste rich in antioxidants.

Choosing whole-wheat pita bread can get many benefits of added fiber, such as slower digestion and added micronutrients.

Serving Size: 4

Prep and Cook Time: 20 min.

INGREDIENTS

- ¾ tsp. kosher salt, divided
- ½ tsp. paprika
- ¾ tsp. black pepper, divided
- ½ tsp. dried oregano
- 1 Tbsp. fresh lemon juice
- Cooking spray
- ⅓ cup thinly sliced red onion
- 3 Tbsp. tahini (sesame seed paste)
- 1 lb. boneless, skinless chicken breasts
- 1 tsp. finely chopped capers
- 1 tsp. Dijon mustard
- ½ tsp. granulated garlic or garlic powder
- 1 cup canned chickpeas, rinsed and drained
- 4 cups chopped romaine lettuce
- 4 (3-oz.) whole-grain pita pockets, sliced in half

Nutrition Information

Per serving: *506 Calories; 12g Fat; 2g Saturated Fat; 83mg Cholesterol; 1082mg Sodium; 63g Carbohydrate; 10g Fiber; 40g Protein; 4g Sugar; 81mg Calcium; 5mg Iron; 826mg Potassium*

DIRECTIONS

STEP 1

Season the chicken wholly with ½ tsp. salt, ½ tsp. black pepper, oregano, and paprika.

STEP 2

Heat a grill pan over medium-high temperature. Use cooking spray to coat pan and chicken breasts. Put the chicken; cook for 5 minutes on each side or until done. Remove cooked chicken from pan; let cool for 5 minutes. Slice chicken thinly across the grain.

STEP 3

Afterwards, prepare Tahini-Caesar dressing by combining tahini, lemon juice, capers, mustard, garlic, and remaining ¼ tsp. each salt and black pepper. Slowly whisk in up to 3 Tbsp. warm water and mixed until smooth.

STEP 4

Add lettuce, red onion, and chickpeas in a sizeable bowl; toss with half of Tahini-Caesar dressing. Divide the lettuce mixture and chicken equally among pita halves; sprinkle on each stuffed pita with remaining Tahini Caesar dressing.

Butternut Squash Soup with Lemongrass

Low FODMAP soup can help the belly heal. When ulcerative colitis attacks, peeled, cooked and mixed vegetables are easy to digest. This soothing soup also provides anti-inflammatory compounds through turmeric and ginger.

Serving Size: 4

Prep and Cook Time: 1 hr.

INGREDIENTS

- ½ tsp. kosher salt
- ½ tsp. ground turmeric
- 1 Tbsp. minced fresh ginger
- 2 Tbsp. extra-virgin olive oil
- 4 cups lower-sodium vegetable broth
- 4 cups peeled and cubed butternut squash
- Microgreens or fresh basil for garnish (optional)
- 2 ½ cups chopped carrots (about 3 large carrots)
- 1 Tbsp. lemongrass paste (find it in tubes near the fresh-herb case)
- ½ cup plus 4 tsp. coconut-milk yogurt, divided (or use the same amount canned coconut milk)

Nutrition Information

Per Serving: *226 Calories; 9g Fat; 2g Saturated Fat; 3mg Cholesterol; 556mg Sodium; 32g Carbohydrate; 6g Fiber; 5g Protein; 12g Sugar; 143mg Calcium; 2mg Iron; 753mg Potassium*

DIRECTIONS

STEP 1

Preheat oil in a Dutch oven or sizeable stockpot over medium heat. Add squash and carrots; cook and stir occasionally for 5 minutes, until lightly golden. Add ginger, lemongrass paste, turmeric, and salt; cook for 2 minutes, until aromatic.

STEP 2

Add broth and increase heat to high. Allow mixture to boil, and then reduce heat to medium-low, cover and cook, for 25 minutes, or until vegetables are tender.

STEP 3

Gently pour the mixture into the blender; add a cup of yogurt. Remove the central part of the blender cover (so that the steam can escape); fix the cover on the blender. Put a clean towel on the opening of the lid. Processing until smooth.

STEP 4

Divide soup equally into 6 serving plates. Swirl 1 tsp. yogurt into each serving, and garnish with fresh basil or microgreens, if needed.

Fried Rice with Miso-Turmeric Vinaigrette

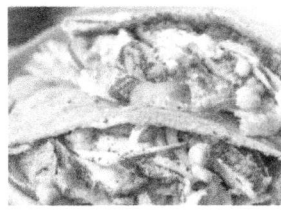 White rice has lower fiber content than brown, so when you're UC symptoms occur, white rice is easier to digest. The dressing provides anti-inflammatory compounds of turmeric and ginger, as well as probiotics that taste miso, to help restore intestinal bacteria.

Serving Size: 4

Prep and Cook Time: 20 min.

INGREDIENTS

- 2 Tbsp. unseasoned rice vinegar
- 1 cup matchstick carrots
- 2 Tbsp. sesame oil (not toasted)
- 2 Tbsp. vegetable oil
- 2 tsp. white miso paste
- ½ tsp. freshly grated ginger
- 3 large eggs, whisked
- ¼ tsp. ground turmeric

- 2 cups roughly chopped baby bok choy
- 2 ½ cups cooked white rice
- 2 Tbsp. lower-sodium soy sauce
- 2 Tbsp. chopped fresh basil

Nutrition Information

Per serving: *322 Calories; 18g Fat; 3g Saturated Fat; 140mg Cholesterol; 443mg Sodium; 32g Carbohydrate; 1g Fiber; 9g Protein; 2g Sugar; 68mg Calcium; 2mg Iron; 92mg Potassium*

DIRECTIONS

STEP 1

Prepare sauce by mixing the vinegar, sesame oil, miso, ginger, and turmeric in a small container; stir with a whisk. Set aside.

STEP 2

Heat vegetable oil in a sizeable skillet over medium-high temperature. Add bok choy and carrots; cook for 5 minutes, stirring occasionally, until tender. Pour in the rice and soy sauce, and press rice down evenly in the skillet. Cook all through, until bottom of rice begins to crisp, about 3 minutes. Toss to combine.

STEP 3

Push the rice and vegetables to all sides, opening a large opening in the center of the pot. Pour in the eggs and beat them thoroughly, until the eggs are messed up, about 1 to 2 minutes. Mix the egg and rice mixture well, then stir in the basil.

STEP 4

Distribute fried rice equally between each of 4 serving plates. Sprinkle Miso Turmeric Vinaigrette on top.

Greek Chicken Pasta Salad

This salad is basically a bowl of Med. diet. This fresh pasta salad is enough for your dinner! Patients with ulcerative colitis who adhere to a Mediterranean diet rich in anti-inflammatory foods may have fewer attacks. Since ingredients such as olive oil and olives provide antioxidant polyphenol plus lean protein and vegetables.

Serving Size: 6

Prep and Cook Time: 30 min.

INGREDIENTS

- 1 lb. boneless, skinless chicken breasts
- ½ tsp. paprika
- 1 tsp. kosher salt, divided
- ½ tsp. black pepper
- Cooking spray

- 12 oz. dry fusilli or rotini pasta
- 2 tsp. minced fresh garlic
- 2 tsp. Dijon mustard
- 4 cups fresh baby spinach
- 2 Tbsp. red wine vinegar
- ¼ cup extra-virgin olive oil
- 1-pint cherry tomatoes, halved
- 1 (14-oz.) can artichoke hearts, drained
- 1 Tbsp. finely chopped fresh oregano
- 1 (2.25-oz.) can sliced black olives, drained
- ½ cup crumbled feta cheese (optional)

Nutrition Information

Per serving: *465 Calories; 14g Fat; 2g Saturated Fat; 55mg Cholesterol; 913mg Sodium; 54g Carbohydrate; 5g Fiber; 28g Protein; 4g Sugar; 59mg Calcium; 4mg Iron; 462mg Potassium*

DIRECTIONS

STEP 1

Season the chicken evenly with a teaspoon of salt, black pepper and chili powder. Heat the grill pan over medium high heat. Coat the pan and chicken breast with cooking spray. Add chicken; cook for 5 minutes on each side or until cooked through. Remove the chicken from the pan; let it cool for 5 minutes. Cut the chicken into small pieces.

STEP 2

Afterwards, according to the package instructions, cook the pasta in salty water and cook until it's cooked. Drain the water and rinse with cold water.

STEP 3

Meanwhile, mix the garlic, mustard, red wine vinegar, oregano and remaining ½ tsp. salt in a bowl; mix with a whisk. Gradually stream in olive oil, whisking often, until combined.

STEP 4

Then, put the tomatoes, spinach, artichoke hearts and black olives into the pasta bowl; stir well. Add chicken, feta and seasoning; toss it up.

Sweet Potato and Lentil Soup

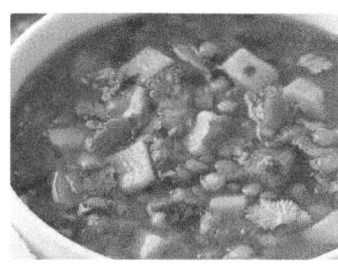
When UC is relieved, beans (such as lentils) can provide you with the ideal fiber and protein dosage. You will also get β-carotene (the precursor of vitamin A) from sweet potatoes.

Serving Size: 6

Prep and Cook Time: 50 min.

INGREDIENTS

- 2 Tbsp. extra-virgin olive oil
- 3 garlic cloves
- 1 cup chopped yellow onion
- 2 Tbsp. tomato paste
- 2 tsp. garam masala
- 1 tsp. kosher salt
- 2 tsp. ground cumin
- 4 cups lower-sodium vegetable broth
- 2 cups water
- 1 (14.5-oz.) can fire-roasted tomatoes
- 1 large sweet potato, peeled and cut into ½-in. pieces (about 2 cups)
- 1 cup uncooked brown lentils
- 1 bunch Lacinato kale, stemmed and roughly chopped
  Fresh parsley for garnish (optional)

Nutrition Information

Per serving: *254 Calories; 6g Fat; 1g Saturated Fat; 0mg Cholesterol; 652mg Sodium; 21g Carbohydrate; 4g Fiber; 12g Protein; 8g Sugar; 125mg Calcium; 6mg Iron; 612mg Potassium*

DIRECTIONS

STEP 1

Heat the oil over medium heat in a sizeable saucepan or Dutch oven. Add onions; cook for 5 minutes, until tender. Add garlic, tomato paste, cumin and garam masala; cook for 2 minutes, stirring occasionally. Add sweet potatoes; stir and cook for 5 minutes. Add the lentils.

STEP 2

Add broth, water, salt and tomatoes; allow the mixture to boil. Reduce the heat, simmer on low heat, and cover until the lentils are cooked and the sweet potatoes are tender, about 30 to 35 minutes. Pour in the kale and stir and cook until the kale is wilted for about 2 minutes.

STEP 3

Divide equally into 6 serving. If needed, you can garnish with fresh parsley.

Quinoa Taco Salads with Chili-Lime Vinaigrette

You will never miss the meat in this vegan vegetable taco salad. Some studies have pointed out that high-fat red meat may cause symptoms of UC. Therefore, this taco salad replaces ground beef (which is high in saturated fat). It uses zesty-spicy quinoa, which is a thin source of plant-based protein.

Serving Size: 4

Prep and Cook Time: 45 min.

INGREDIENTS

- 1 cup lower-sodium vegetable broth
- 2 tsp. prepared taco seasoning
- 1 tsp. lime zest, plus 2 Tbsp. fresh lime juice (separate)
- ½ tsp. chili powder
- ½ cup dry quinoa, well rinsed
- ½ tsp. kosher salt, divided
- 1 ½ tsp. pure maple syrup
- ¼ cup extra-virgin olive oil
- 8 cups chopped romaine lettuce
- 1 ripe avocado, well sliced
- 1 cup frozen fire-roasted corn, thawed
- 1-pint cherry tomatoes, halved
- 1 (15-oz.) can black beans, well rinsed and drained
- ⅓ cup thinly sliced red onion

Nutrition Information

Perserving: *374 Calories; 23g Fat; 3g Saturated Fat; 0mg Cholesterol; 704mg Sodium; 37g Carbohydrate; 12g Fiber; 9g Protein; 6g Sugar; 92mg Calcium; 3mg Iron; 768mg Potassium*

DIRECTIONS

STEP 1

Combine the quinoa, broth, and taco seasoning in a small pot over medium high heat; bring to a boil. Cover the lid, reduce the heat to low-medium level, and simmer until the soup is absorbed, about 15 minutes. Remove from the heat; stand up, cover the pot, let it sit for 15 minutes, then fluff it with a fork. Put it in a bowl and transfer to the refrigerator to cool.

STEP 2

While waiting, mix the lime zest and juice, chili powder, ¼ tsp. salt, and maple syrup in a small bowl; stir well using whisk. Carefully stream in oil, whisking continuously, until combined.

STEP 3

Place lettuce, black beans, corn, onions, tomatoes and the remaining teaspoons of salt in a large bowl; toss it up. Distribute equally among four bowls. Remove the quinoa from the refrigerator and spoon equally on the salad. Drizzle chili lime balsamic vinegar on top and sprinkle sliced avocado on each salad.

Tuna Niçoise Grain Bowl

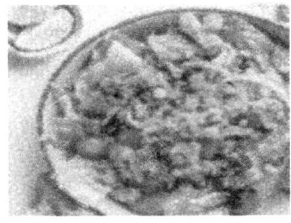

During the remission period, patients with ulcerative colitis are encouraged to follow the Mediterranean diet, focusing on fish rich in omega 3, such as salmon and tuna, as well as whole grains, olive oil and fresh produce. This full bowl has everything and more.

Serving Size: 4

Prep and Cook Time: 40 min.

INGREDIENTS

- 2 tsp. honey
- 1 cup dry farro, rinsed
- ½ tsp. kosher salt, divided
- 12 oz. small red or fingerling potatoes
- 6 oz. haricots verts (French green beans)
- 2 Tbsp. fresh lemon juice
- 2 tsp. chopped fresh oregano or ¾ tsp. dried
- 1 tsp. Dijon mustard
- ¼ tsp. black pepper
- ¼ cup extra-virgin olive oil
- 2 oz. black or green olives, sliced
- 1 cup halved cherry tomatoes
- 2 (5-oz.) cans tuna, drained and flaked
- 2 soft-boiled eggs, halved (optional)

Nutrition Information

Per serving: *489 Calories; 19g Fat; 3g Saturated Fat; 30mg Cholesterol; 688mg Sodium; 30mg Carbohydrate; 6g Fiber;*

26g Protein; 7g Sugar; 81mg Calcium; 3mg Iron; 814mg Potassium

DIRECTIONS

STEP 1

Place farro in a small saucepan; add ¼ tsp. salt and 3 cups water. Allow to boil; lower the heat to medium-low, and simmer, with the lid covered, for 30 minutes. Drain any excess liquid.

STEP 2

Meanwhile, Place the potatoes in a separate large pot; add water to cover 2 inches. Bring to a high boil; reduce to medium-low level, then cook for 15 minutes. Add the haricots; cook for another 6 minutes. Drain and rinse the potatoes and haricots. Cut the potatoes into halves or quarters according to their size. Set aside.

STEP 3

Place the lemon juice, oregano, honey, mustard, remaining salt and black pepper in a small bowl; stir to combine. Gradually infuse olive oil, stirring constantly until smooth.

STEP 4

Divide the cooked farro, potatoes, haricots, tomatoes, tuna and olives evenly into four bowls. Add half an egg to each bowl, then drizzle the dressing on top.

Lemony Orzo Salad with Flaked Salmon

Simple pasta with salmon rich in omega can soothe an angry belly. It looks a bit like rice, but orzo is actually a short-cut white pasta that has low fiber content and is easy in the belly of UC patients. Salmon provides omega-3 fatty acids EPA and DHA, which can help relieve systemic inflammation.

Serving Size: 4

Prep and Cook Time: 45 min.

INGREDIENTS

- 1 cup uncooked orzo
- 2 cups lower-sodium vegetable broth
- ½ tsp. kosher salt, divided
- ¼ tsp. black pepper
- 2 cups fresh baby spinach
- 1 Tbsp. fresh lemon juice
- 2 (6-oz.) center-cut salmon fillets
- ⅓ cup sun-dried tomatoes packed in oil, plus 2 Tbsp. oil from jar, divided
- 2 Tbsp. fresh parsley leaves

Nutrition Information

Perserving: *374 Calories; 14g Fat; 2g Saturated Fat; 47mg Cholesterol; 395mg Sodium; 37g Carbohydrate; 3g Fiber; 23g Protein; 3g Sugar; 55mg Calcium; 2mg Iron; 571mg Potassium*

DIRECTIONS

STEP 1

Heat 1 tablespoon the sun-dried tomato oil medium -sized pot, over high heat. Add orzo; cook for 2 minutes, stirring often. Add broth and teaspoon salt; allow to boil. Cover the pot, reduce the heat, and simmer for 10 to 12 minutes, or until the broth is absorbed.

STEP2

Remove the pan from the heat; leave covered for 5 minutes. Stir in spinach, sun-dried tomatoes and lemon juice (spinach will wilt quickly).

STEP 3

At the same time, preheat the broiler with an oven rack 6 inches from the heat. Brush salmon with 1 tablespoon of sun-dried tomato oil and season with the remaining teaspoon salt and black pepper. Place the fillets (face down) on a foil-lined baking sheet. Broil to your desire, for 8 to 10 minutes. Use a metal spatula to remove the fillets from the foil.

STEP 4

Take away the salmon skin; use a fork to gradually pull the flesh into large flakes; toss with orzo. Divide orzo salad evenly among 4 plates; serve with fresh parsley.

Zucchini Noodles

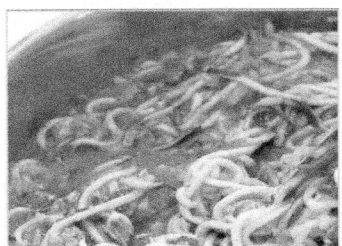

It is smart to avoid eating high-fiber vegetables during flares, and cooked zucchini noodles are an excellent alternative for low residues. (By the way, low residue means low fiber.) The tofu here is an important source of calcium, which is especially important for UC patients on steroids.

Serving Size: 4

Prep and Cook Time: 20 min.

INGREDIENTS

- 3 Tbsp. natural creamy peanut butter
- Juice of 1 lime
- 2 Tbsp. lower-sodium soy sauce
- 1 ½ tsp. freshly grated ginger
- 2 tsp. pure maple syrup
- 1 red bell pepper, thinly sliced
- 2 Tbsp. extra-virgin olive oil, divided
- 1 ½ cups matchstick carrots

- 1 (14-oz.) block extra-firm tofu, drained, patted dry, and cut into 1-in.
  cubes
- ½ tsp. kosher salt, divided
- 4 medium zucchinis, trimmed and spiralized into thin noodles

Nutrition Information

Perserving: *311 Calories; 19g Fat; 3g Saturated Fat; 0mg Cholesterol; 591mg*
Sodium; 20g Carbohydrate; 5g Fiber; 17g Protein; 11g Sugar; 126mg Calcium; 3mg Iron; 661mg Potassium

DIRECTIONS

STEP 1

In a small bowl, mix together peanut butter, soy sauce, ginger, lime juice and maple syrup and mix well.

STEP 2

Heat 1 tablespoon oil in a medium nonstick pan. Add tofu; cook for 8 to 10 minutes, or until the tofu is golden and crisp, stirring once a while. Season the tofu with a small ¼ teaspoon salt; transfer to a plate.

STEP 3

Add the remaining 1 tablespoon oil into the pan. Boil the carrots and bell peppers until tender, about 5 to 6 minutes, stirring occasionally. Season with the remaining ¼ teaspoon salt.

STEP 4

Put the zucchini noodles in the pot; cook for 2 to 3 minutes, turning frequently to heat, but not fully cooked. Add the tofu and half of the peanut butter to the frying pan. Toss to combine.

STEP 5

Distribute the zucchini noodle mixture evenly on 4 plates. Drizzle the remaining peanut sauce on top.

DINNERS RECIPES

Seared Scallops with Avocado-Citrus Salsa

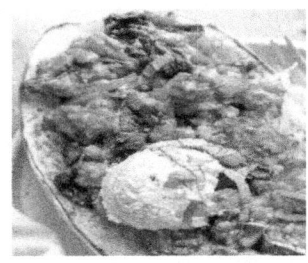 Fruits like avocado and orange are low in roughage and easier to digest when UC symptoms are flaring up. They're also rich in vitamin C, which can enhance iron absorption (especially important if your UC is contributing to anemia).

Serving Size: 4

Prep and Cook Time: 30 min.

INGREDIENTS

- ¾ cup dry quinoa, rinsed
- 1 lb. sea scallops, patted dry
- 2 cups lower-sodium vegetable broth ?2 Tbsp. extra-virgin olive oil
- 1 cup diced avocado (from 1 avocado)
- ¾ tsp. kosher salt, divided
- ½ tsp. black pepper, divided
- 2 Tbsp. chopped fresh parsley
- ¾ cup peeled and diced orange segments
- ¼ cup finely chopped red bell pepper
- 1 tsp. orange zest, plus 2 Tbsp. fresh orange juice

Nutrition Information

Per serving: *352 Calories; 15g Fat; 2g Saturated Fat; 27mg Cholesterol;*
880mg Sodium; 35g Carbohydrate; 7g Fiber; 19g Protein; 6g Sugar; 58mg
Calcium; 3mg Iron; 702mg Potassium

DIRECTIONS

STEP 1

In a small pan, mix the quinoa and broth and bring it to a boil. Reduce the heat to minimum, cover and simmer for about 15 minutes, until most of the broth is absorbed. Fluff quinoa using a fork and cover to keep warm.

STEP 2

Meanwhile, heat 1 Tbsp. oil in a sizeable skillet over medium-high. Drizzle scallops with ½ tsp. salt and ¼ tsp. black pepper. Add scallops to pan; cook 2 minutes. Flip and cook for 2 additional minutes or until the degree of doneness is achieved. Remove the scallops from pan and keep warm.

STEP 3

Mix the orange, avocado, segments, bell pepper, orange zest and juice, remaining 1 Tbsp. oil, ¼ tsp. salt, and ¼ tsp. black pepper in a bowl; slowly mix them up to combine.

STEP 4

Serve the quinoa and scallops equally between four serving plates. Top with Avocado-Citrus Salsa, and garnish with fresh parsley.

Spaghetti Squash Lasagna Boats with Almond Ricotta

When you have ulcerative colitis, fatty ground beef and milk can worsen the symptoms. This recipe uses lean ground turkey breast and faux-ricotta cheese made of blanched almonds as an alternative.

Serving Size: 4

Prep and Cook Time: 1 hr.

INGREDIENTS

- 2 medium spaghetti squashes
- 1 lb. ground turkey breast
- ⅓ cup warm water
- 2 cups fresh baby spinach
- ¾ tsp. kosher salt, divided
- 1 (15-oz.) can crushed tomatoes
- 1 tsp. nutritional yeast
- ¾ cup blanched almonds
- 2 Tbsp. extra-virgin olive oil, divided
- 2 tsp. fresh lemon juice
- 4 Tbsp. fresh chopped basil leaves, divided

Nutrition Information

Per serving: *456 Calories; 23g Fat; 3g Saturated Fat; 55mg Cholesterol; 709mg Sodium; 30g Carbohydrate; 9g Fiber; 37g Protein; 12g Sugar; 181mg Calcium; 5mg Iron; 782mg Potassium*

DIRECTIONS

STEP 1

Preheat the oven to 400°F. Cut the squashes, lengthwise, in half and extract the seeds. Rub the flesh with 1 Tbsp. of oil, and position on a rimmed baking sheet, cut side down. Bake for 40 minutes, or until the flesh is soft.

STEP 2

After that, heat the remaining 1 Tbsp. oil in a sizeable skillet over medium heat. Add the turkey; cook for 6 to 7 minutes, or until fully cooked, breaking the meat into small pieces. Stir in the spinach; cook, until wilted, for 2 minutes. Season with ½ tsp. salt.

STEP 3

Pour in tomatoes and 2 Tbsp. of basil; lower the heat. Cover to keep it warm.

STEP 4

Combine the lemon juice, almonds, nutritional yeast, water, and the remaining ¼ tsp. salt in a high-power food processor or blender. Blend until perfectly smooth.

STEP 5

Remove the spaghetti squash from the oven and shred flesh (like strands) on the spaghetti using a fork.

STEP 6

Place on each squash half with the turkey mixture. Top with 2 Tbsp. Almond Ricotta. Serve evenly with remaining 2 Tbsp. basil.

Sheet-Pan Salmon Romesco with Green Beans & Crushed Potatoes

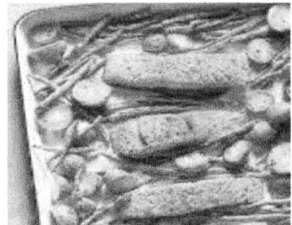 It takes only 15 minutes to prepare this easy-to-digest meal. Steer clear of high-fibre vegetables during a flare, which may worsen an already-irritated colon. Better alternatives include cooked green beans and potatoes that are naturally poor in FODMAPs. Discomfort or bloating is the last thing you need when you have UC.

Serving Size: 4

Prep and Cook Time: 45 min.

INGREDIENTS

- 12 oz. baby yellow potatoes
- 1 lb. skin-on salmon, sliced into 4 fillets
- ¼ cup walnuts
- 1 tsp. kosher salt, divided
- ¾ tsp. black pepper, divided
- ¼ tsp. paprika
- 8 oz. haricots verts (French green beans)
- ¾ cup jarred roasted red peppers, drained
- 2 Tbsp. plus 2 tsp. extra-virgin olive oil, divided
- 2 tsp. fresh lemon juice
- Fresh parsley for garnish (optional)

Nutrition Information

Per serving: *376 Calories; 21g Fat; 3g Saturated Fat; 62mg Cholesterol;*
781mg Sodium; 23g Carbohydrate; 4g Fiber; 26g Protein; 4g Sugar; 105mg Calcium; 3mg Iron; 715mg Potassium

DIRECTIONS

STEP 1

Preheat the oven to 425°F.

STEP 2

Put the potatoes in a small saucepan; containing water, boil and simmer for 12 minutes, or until almost tender. Drain the water.

STEP 3

Coat a baking sheet using a parchment paper; place salmon fillets on one side. Rub the salmon with 1 Tbsp. of the oil, and sprinkle on ¼ tsp. Black pepper and ¼ tsp. salt. Keep the potatoes next to salmon. With the flat side of a measuring cup, gently crush the potatoes, brush potatoes thoroughly with 1 Tbsp. oil, and drizzle on ¼ tsp. salt, and ¼ tsp. black pepper. Place the pan in the oven and bake for 8 minutes.

STEP 4

Remove the pan from the oven and add the haricots verts to the baking sheet to open space. Toss with 2 tsp. oil and ¼ tsp. salt. Put it back in the oven for another 8 minutes. Switch the broiler to high; broil until the salmon and potatoes are browned, about 2 minutes.

STEP 5

Combine the red peppers, walnuts, paprika, lemon juice, and the remaining ¼ tsp. salt and ¼ tsp. In a food processor or blender, add black pepper; blend until smooth.

STEP 6

Spoon Romesco over the potatoes and salmon fillets. Garnish with fresh parsley, if needed.

Sesame-Seared Tuna Steaks with Soba Noodles

Swap in booming inflammation-fighting seafood steaks for beef a couple times a week. UC wreaks its most obvious havoc in your colon, but UC is actually a systemic inflammatory disease that can affect your entire body. Omega-3-rich seafood like tuna will help turn down the heat. it takes minutes to prepare. **Serving Size:** 4 **Prep and Cook Time:** 20 min.

INGREDIENTS

- 8 oz. soba (Japanese buckwheat noodles)
- 2 Tbsp. sweet chili sauce
- 1 (6-oz.) bag snow peas
- 2 Tbsp. fresh lime juice
- ¼ cup lower-sodium soy sauce
- 2 Tbsp. light sesame oil
- ¼ cup fresh cilantro leaves
- 1 Tbsp. vegetable oil
- ½ tsp. kosher salt
- 2 Tbsp. white sesame seeds
- 2 Tbsp. black sesame seeds
- 2 (8-oz.) ahi tuna steaks
- Cooking spray
- 2 Tbsp. thinly sliced green onion

Nutrition Information

Per serving: *483 Calories; 16g Fat; 2g Saturated Fat; 40mg Cholesterol; 1342mg Sodium; 49g Carbohydrate; 2g Fiber; 40g Protein; 2g Sugar; 136mg Calcium; 5mg Iron; 707mg Potassium*

DIRECTIONS

STEP 1

Cook the soba noodles according to package instructions. Add the snow peas in the final 3 minutes. Rinse with warm water and drain well.

STEP 2

Mix the lime juice, soy sauce, chili sauce, and sesame oil in a sizeable bowl; stir well. Add the soba mixture and cilantro; toss to combine.

STEP 3

Put the white sesame and black sesame in a shallow dish. Coat the tuna steak with cooking spray and sprinkle with salt evenly. Coat both sides of each steak with sesame seeds and press lightly to make it adhere.

Step 4

Heat the vegetable oil in a large frying pan to medium high. Pour the tuna into the pot; cook for 3 minutes on each side to reach a moderately rare or cooked level. Cut the tuna into thin slices.

STEP 5

Divide the soba mixture evenly into four plates. Top with 4 ounces of tuna and garnished with chopped green onion.

Note: If sesame seeds trigger your UC symptoms, you can skip it. This dish is still delicious!

Red Curry Chicken and Rice

Mild spices and white rice can be soothing. When symptoms of UC appear, prepare this relaxing dish. Spice blends such as curry powder can enhance flavor without adding extra fat, salt or trigger food during UC outbreaks. Chopped chicken breasts and peeled cooked potatoes are also easy to digest.

Serving Size: 6

Prep and Cook Time: 40 min.

INGREDIENTS

- 1 Tbsp. curry powder
- 2 Tbsp. extra-virgin olive oil
- 2 tsp. freshly grated ginger
- 1 tsp. paprika
- 1 (14.5-oz.) can diced tomatoes
- 2 cups peeled and cubed Russet potato (from 1 large potato)
- 3 Tbsp. natural peanut butter
- 2 cups lower-sodium vegetable broth
- ¾ tsp. kosher salt
- ½ tsp. black pepper
- 2 cups fresh baby spinach
- 1 ½ cups shredded rotisserie chicken
- 3 cups cooked white rice for serving
- Fresh basil for garnish, if desired
- 1 ½ cups unsweetened refrigerated cashew milk (or 1 can light coconut milk)

Nutrition Information

Per serving: *333 Calories; 11g Fat; 2g Saturated Fat; 32mg Cholesterol; 628mg Sodium; 40g Carbohydrate; 4g Fiber; 17g Protein; 3g Sugar; 99mg Calcium; 3mg Iron; 538mg Potassium*

DIRECTIONS

STEP 1

Heat oil in a sizeable high-sided skillet over medium heat. Stir in paprika, curry powder and ginger; cook for 2 minutes. Stir in the potatoes and cook for 5 minutes, stirring occasionally, until light golden brown.

STEP 2

Add peanut butter, broth, salt and pepper; allow the mixture to boil. Lower the heat to medium-low, and cover the pot until the potatoes are tender, about 20 minutes.

STEP 3

Put the spinach and cook until it's wilted, about 2 minutes. Put the chicken and cashew milk; stir to combine, leave uncovered and Simmer for 5 minutes.

STEP 4

Put ½ cup rice in each of 6 serving plates and top with 1 cup curry mixture. Serve with fresh basil, if desired.

Moroccan Quinoa-Stuffed Eggplant with Pine-Nut Parmesan

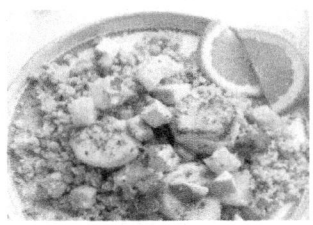 Don't let the mild taste of eggplant fool you. This vegetable is rich in vitamins and minerals. Patients with UC are sensitive to lactose, this recipe uses pine nuts and nutritional yeast to make plant-based Parmesan cheese.

Serving Size: 4

Prep and Cook Time: 1 hr.

INGREDIENTS

- 2 medium eggplants
- 3 garlic cloves, minced
- 3 Tbsp. extra-virgin olive oil, divided
- ¾ tsp. kosher salt, divided
- ½ cup dry quinoa
- 1 (14.5-oz.) can diced tomatoes
- 2 Tbsp. mild harissa paste
- 2 cups lower-sodium vegetable broth
- 1 Tbsp. nutritional yeast
- 3 Tbsp. finely chopped pine nuts (or slivered almonds)
- ¼ tsp. garlic powder
- 4 Tbsp. thinly sliced fresh basil leaves

Nutrition Information

Per serving: 331 Calories; 17g Fat; 2g Saturated Fat; 0mg Cholesterol; 734mg
Sodium; 39g Carbohydrate; 12g Fiber; 8g Protein; 14g Sugar; 89mg Calcium; 2mg Iron; 1023mg Potassium

DIRECTIONS

STEP 1

Preheat the oven to 375°F.

STEP 2

Cut the eggplant in half along the length of the stem. Cut the flesh of the eggplant into a circle, and then dig out the flesh. Set aside. Place the eggplant half face up on the baking sheet.

STEP 3

Brush the eggplant halves with 1 Tbsp. of the olive oil and ¼ tsp of salt. Roast the eggplant for 20 minutes, or until golden brown and lightly tender.

STEP 4

At the same time, heat the remaining 2 tablespoons oil in a sizeable frying pan over medium heat. Chop the reserved eggplant flesh and put it in the pot. Cook for 6 to 7 minutes, until tender. Add garlic, harissa, quinoa and teaspoon salt; cook for 2 minutes, stirring often.

STEP 5

Add the diced tomatoes and broth, and bring the mixture to a boil. Simmer for a short while, cover the pot and cook for 15 to 20 minutes, until the quinoa is cooked and absorbed most of the liquid.

STEP 6

Remove the eggplant halves from the oven and add the quinoa mixture evenly. Place back in the oven for 15 minutes.

STEP 7

Mix pine nuts, nutritional yeast, garlic powder, and remaining ¼ tsp salt in a medium bowl. Drizzle Pine Nut Parmesan over each the eggplant half, and serve each with 1 Tbsp. basil.

Chili Shrimp Tacos with Avocado-Tomatillo Sauce

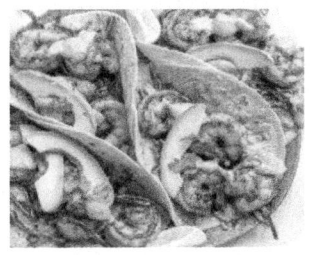

Spice up your tacos with Mediterranean flavor, replace the beef with shrimp. This recipe also contains fiber rich vegetables, which can help feed beneficial intestinal bacteria,   thereby helping   to control symptoms.

Serving Size: 4

Prep and Cook Time: 25 min.

INGREDIENTS

- 1 lb. medium raw shrimp, peeled and deveined
- ½ tsp. ground cumin
- 1 tsp. chili powder
- 1 tsp. kosher salt, divided
- 1 Tbsp. plus 2 tsp. extra-virgin olive oil, divided
- 6 oz. fresh tomatillos, peeled and halved
- 3 Tbsp. thinly sliced green onion
- 1 Tbsp. fresh lime juice
- ⑦1 ripe avocado, divided
- 2 cups shredded red cabbage
- 8 (6-in.) corn tortillas, warmed
- ½ cup fresh cilantro leaves, divided
- ½ medium jalapeño, seeded (optional)

Nutrition Information

Per serving: *344 Calories; 14g Fat; 2g Saturated Fat; 143mg Cholesterol; 670mg Sodium; 33g Carbohydrate; 7g Fiber; 19g Protein; 4g Sugar; 93mg Calcium; 1mg Iron; 589mg Potassium*

DIRECTIONS

STEP 1

Put the shrimp in a small bowl and toss with cumin, chili powder and ½ tsp. salt. Heat 1 Tbsp. oil in a sizeable skillet over medium-high heat.

STEP 2

Place the shrimp into the cooking pan and arrange in a single layer, cook for 3 minutes. Turn other side and cook additional 2 minutes. Transfer to a bowl; keep warm.

STEP 3

To Prepare the Avocado-Tomatillo sauce, mix ½ of the avocado, ¼ cup cilantro, jalapeño (optional), tomatillos and remaining ½ tsp. salt in a blender; blend until smooth.

STEP 4

Put cabbage, remaining ¼ cup cilantro, lime juice, remaining 2 tsp. oil, green onion and ¼ tsp. salt in a bowl; toss to combine.

STEP 5

Distribute the shrimp and cabbage mixture equally between warmed tortillas. Each taco is topped with 2 Tbsp. Avocado-Tomatillo Sauce. Slice and garnish with remaining ½ avocado.

Chicken Piccata Pasta

This dinner is perfect for special occasions and is fast enough to take a dip in a working day. Compared with most Piccata pasta, this pasta can reduce the butter content to keep saturated fat at a low level (a large amount of fat can trigger the occurrence of ulcerative colitis). Enhance specificity and increase antioxidants

Serving Size: 4

Prep and Cook Time: 25 min.

INGREDIENTS

- 3 Tbsp. extra-virgin olive oil
- 10 oz. dry angel hair pasta
- 1 Tbsp. minced fresh garlic (or a tsp. if you're sensitive)
- ¼ cup brined capers, drained
- ⅓ cup chopped fresh parsley
- 3 Tbsp. unsalted butter, divided
- 1 lb. skinless, boneless chicken breasts, butterflied and then cut in half
- ½ tsp. kosher salt
- ¾ tsp. black pepper, divided
- 3 Tbsp. all-purpose flour
- ½ cup dry white wine
- 1 cup lower-sodium chicken broth
- 2 Tbsp. fresh lemon juice

Nutrition Information

Per serving: *623 Calories; 25g Fat; 8g Saturated Fat; 106mg Cholesterol; 519mg Sodium; 59g Carbohydrate; 3g Fiber; 37g Protein; 3g Sugar; 39mg Calcium; 3mg Iron; 617mg Potassium*

DIRECTIONS

STEP 1

According to package directions, cook the pasta in boiling salted water until hardened. Drain the water and transfer to a plate.

STEP 2

Heat oil and 2 Tbsp. butter at the same time in the large frying pan over medium-high heat. Season the chicken with salt and ½ tsp. black pepper.
Sprinkle flour evenly and shake off excess flour. Add the chicken to the frying pan and cook without disturbing for 3 minutes per side, until golden brown. Transfer to a plate.

STEP 3

Pour the garlic into the pot; cook for 1 minute, stirring constantly. Add wine; cook for 2 minutes, scrape the brown bits from the pan, until halved. Stir in the broth, lemon juice, capers and the remaining teaspoon. Black pepper. Put the chicken back in the pot and simmer for 5 minutes.

STEP 4

Remove the chicken from the pot and place it on the pasta. Add the remaining 1 tbsp. butter into the pan and stir vigorously to mix.

STEP 5

Drizzle sauce over chicken and pasta. Serve with fresh parsley.

Note: Garlic is a high-FODMAP

Balsamic-Roasted Salmon with Artichoke Gremolata

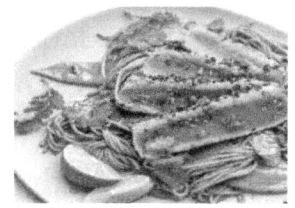 This dish is restaurant-worthy, a cinch to make, and packed with ingredients that are UC remission-friendly. For good reason, salmon is considered a superfood: it is a rich source of vitamin D, which can help quench inflammation in the intestines.

Serving Size: 4

Prep and Cook Time: 50 min.

INGREDIENTS

- 4 (6-oz.) salmon fillets
- ½ tsp. kosher salt

- 2 Tbsp. balsamic vinegar
- 3 Tbsp. extra-virgin olive oil, divided
- 2 tsp. Dijon mustard
- 2 tsp. honey
- ¾ cup halved cherry tomatoes
- ½ cup canned artichoke hearts in brine, finely chopped
- 1 Tbsp. finely chopped pine nuts (or raw slivered almonds)
- 2 cups fresh spinach
- 1 garlic clove, minced
- 1 Tbsp. fresh lemon juice
- 2 Tbsp. fresh chopped parsley
- ½ tsp. black pepper
- 2 cups lower-sodium vegetable broth
- 1 ⅓ cup dry pearl couscous

Nutrition Information

Per serving: *634 Calories; 23g Fat; 3g Saturated Fat; 94mg Cholesterol; 534mg Sodium; 64g Carbohydrate; 4g Fiber; 44g Protein; 7g Sugar; 68mg Calcium; 3mg Iron; 912mg Potassium*

DIRECTIONS

STEP 1

In a wide-rimmed bowl, put the salmon and season with salt. Mix 1 tbsp. oil, vinegar, mustard, and honey in a medium sized bowl turn with a whisk. Set aside 2 tbsp., pour the remaining mixture over the salmon and leave to stand for 15 minutes.

STEP 2

In the meantime, combine the artichokes, pine nuts, garlic, lemon juice, black pepper, parsley, and the remaining 2 Tbsp. olive oil in a bowl; blend well. Only set aside.

STEP 3

In a medium saucepan, bring the broth to a boil. Add couscous, lower the heat to a simmer, cover and cook for around 15 minutes until tender. Remove from the heat and stir in the tomatoes and spinach. Cover to keep warm.

STEP 4

Preheat the oven to 450°F. Insert the salmon on a baking sheet lined with foil and bake it for 8 minutes. Remove from the oven and brush with reserved marinade; put back in the oven, and bake for additional 5 minutes.

STEP 5

Divide the couscous mixture equally into 4 bowls each. Serve each bowl with 1 salmon fillet and 2 Tbsp. artichoke gremolata. Mild spices and white rice satisfy and help relax. Any time UC symptoms flare up, serve this comforting dish.

Red Curry Chicken and Rice

Soft Spice blends like curry powder boost taste without adding extra fat, salt, or trigger foods during a UC flare. Crushed chicken breast and peeled, cooked potato is also easy on digestion.

Serving Size: 6

Prep and Cook Time: 40 min.

INGREDIENTS

- 2 Tbsp. extra-virgin olive oil
- 1 Tbsp. curry powder
- 2 cups lower-sodium vegetable broth
- 2 tsp. freshly grated ginger
- 1 tsp. paprika
- 2 cups peeled and cubed Russet potato (from 1 large potato)
- 3 Tbsp. natural peanut butter
- 1 (14.5-oz.) can diced tomatoes
- ¾ tsp. kosher salt
- ½ tsp. black pepper
- 2 cups fresh baby spinach
- 1 ½ cups shredded rotisserie chicken
- 3 cups cooked white rice for serving

- 1 ½ cups unsweetened refrigerated cashew milk (or 1 can light coconut milk)
- Fresh basil for garnish, if desired

Nutrition Information

Per serving: *323 Calories; 11g Fat; 2g Saturated Fat; 32mg Cholesterol; 628mg Sodium; 40g Carbohydrate; 4g Fiber; 17g Protein; 3g Sugar; 99mg Calcium; 3mg Iron; 518mg Potassium*

DIRECTIONS

STEP 1

Heat oil to medium in a big, high-sided skillet. Insert curry powder, paprika, and ginger; cook for 2 minutes. Stir in the potatoes and cook for 5 minutes, stirring occasionally, until golden brown. Insert peanut butter, broth, tomatoes, salt, and pepper; bring the mixture to a boil.

STEP 2

Reduce to medium-low and simmer, covered, for about 20 minutes, or until the potato is tender. Stir in the spinach and cook for about 2 minutes, until wilted. Add the cashew milk and chicken; stir to mix. for 5 minutes, uncovered.

STEP 3

Put ½ cup rice in each of 6 bowls, top with 1 cup curry mixture. Serve with fresh basil, if needed.

SNACKS AND DESSERTS RECIPES

Cherry Almond-Butter Bars

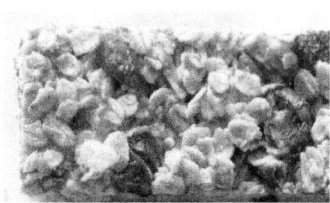 These protein and fiber-packed bars beat the packed bars every day of the week. Who knew you could get an increase in calcium from almonds and pecans? This is a big advantage for people with UC who are often deficient in minerals. These bars also provide heart-healthy fat and dietary fiber.

Serving Size: 10

Prep and Cook Time: 35 min.

INGREDIENTS

- ¾ cup creamy almond butter
- 1 tsp. vanilla extract
- ½ tsp. kosher salt
- ⅓ cup pecans
- 1 egg white, whisked
- 2 cups old-fashioned oats

- ¼ cup pure maple syrup
- ½ cup chopped dried cherries

Nutrition Information

Per serving: 243 Calories; 14g Fat; 2g Saturated Fat; 0mg Cholesterol; 147mg
Sodium; 27g Carbohydrate; 5g Fiber; 7g Protein; 11g Sugar; 95mg Calcium; 2mg Iron; 258mg Potassium

DIRECTIONS

STEP 1

Preheat the oven to 350°F. Arrange an 8x8-inch square baking pan with parchment paper.

STEP 2

Mix the almond butter, vanilla, maple syrup, salt and egg white in a large bowl; stir to combine. Stir in the oats, cherries and pistachios, then transfer the mixture to the prepared baking pan. Use a spatula to press the mixture firmly into the pan.

STEP 3

Bake for 20 minutes, or until it turns light brown. Allow it cool completely before removing it from the pan using parchment paper. Place on a cutting board and cut into 10 bars.

Strawberry-Banana Nice Cream

Homemade ice cream will not cause abdominal pain. When the colon is stimulated, bananas are easy to digest, and the potassium content in bananas is high, which is one of the electrolytes lost in diarrhea caused by flare.

Serving Size: 2

Prep and Cook Time: 10 min.

INGREDIENTS

- 1 cup frozen strawberries
- 1 ½ medium frozen bananas, chopped
- 3 Tbsp. unsweetened vanilla almond milk

Nutrition Information

Per serving: *107 Calories; 1g Fat; 0g Saturated Fat; 0mg Cholesterol; 19mg Sodium; 27g Carbohydrate; 4g Fiber; 1g Protein; 14g Sugar; 35mg Calcium; 1mg Iron; 425mg Potassium*

DIRECTION

STEP 1

Mix all ingredients in a high-power mixer. Blend until creamy, stop and scrape off the sides as needed. Enjoy immediately or spread out in a bread pan, freeze for another 30 minutes, then remove with an ice cream scoop.

Chocolate-Avocado Mousse

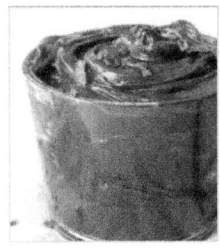 The healthy ingredients of this mousse incorporate a nutritious and easily tolerated avocado, which is also an important source of potassium. A dessert you that can make you feel better when you have UC flare; it's dairy-free with healthy fats.

Serving Size: 4

Prep and Cook Time: 1 hr. 10 min.

INGREDIENTS

- 2 large ripe avocados
- ¼ cup pure maple syrup
- ¼ cup regular unsweetened cocoa powder
- 1 tsp. vanilla extract
- 2 Tbsp. dark baking cocoa
- 3 Tbsp. unsweetened cashew milk (or unsweetened almond, coconut, or soy milk)
- ¼ tsp. sea salt

- Fresh raspberries for garnish (optional)

Nutrition Information

Per serving: *212 Calories; 16g Fat; 3g Saturated Fat; 0mg Cholesterol; 190mg Sodium; 27g Carbohydrate; 9g Fiber; 4g Protein; 13g Sugar; 44mg Calcium; 1mg Iron; 623mg Potassium*

DIRECTION

STEP 1

Put all ingredients (except raspberries) in a high-power blender or food processor; blend until smooth. Transfer to a bowl and let cool for 1 hour. Divide into four bowls; top with the raspberries.

Rosemary Roasted-Chickpea Snack Mix

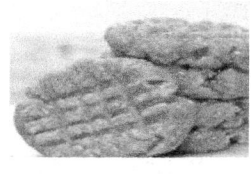 Chickpeas contain fiber, protein and a lot of nutrients. Chickpeas are small power plants of protein and fiber, exactly what you want in a snack.

Serving Size: 6

Prep and Cook Time: 1 hr.

INGREDIENTS

- 1 tsp. kosher salt
- 1 (15-oz.) can chickpeas, drained, rinsed, and patted dried
- ½ cup chopped toasted walnuts
- 1 Tbsp. extra-virgin olive oil
- ½ cup chopped dried apricots
- 1 Tbsp. finely chopped fresh rosemary
- ½ tsp. garlic powder
- ¼ tsp. cayenne pepper

Nutrition Information

Per serving: *204 Calories; 10g Fat; 1g Saturated Fat; 0mg Cholesterol; 473mg Sodium; 25g Carbohydrate; 6g Fiber; 7g Protein; 7g Sugar; 52mg Calcium; 1mg Iron; 124mg Potassium*

DIRECTIONS

STEP 1

Preheat the oven to 400°F. Mix the chickpeas with oil, rosemary, salt, garlic powder and cayenne. Arrange on a framed baking sheet and bake for 45 minutes, or until golden brown and crispy, toss once halfway through. Let it cool on a baking sheet for 10 minutes, then transfer to a bowl.

STEP 2

Add walnuts and apricots to the chickpeas; toss up. Store at room temperature in a closed container for up to 5 days.

Peanut-Butter Cookie-Dough Bites

This treat provides good protein without being overly sweet. During a UC outbreak, smaller, more frequent meals and snacks are usually best. These bites provide enough energy to help you through the difficult times. **Serving Size:** 10

Prep and Cook Time: 15 min.

INGREDIENTS

- 1 ¾ cups old-fashioned rolled oats
- ¼ cup pure maple syrup
- 1 cup natural peanut butter
- 1 tsp. vanilla extract
- ½ tsp. ground cinnamon
- ½ tsp. kosher salt

Nutrition Information

Per serving: *223 Calories; 14g Fat; 2g Saturated Fat; 0mg Cholesterol; 181mg Sodium; 20g Carbohydrate; 3g Fiber; 7g Protein; 6g Sugar; 17mg Calcium; 1mg Iron; 72mg Potassium*

DIRECTIONS

STEP 1

Place the oats in the food processor; process until thoroughly chopped.
Transfer to a large bowl and add the remaining ingredients; stir to combine.

STEP 2

Use a cookie scoop to make the mixture into 20-22 bites, or roll into small balls. Store in an airtight container and refrigerate for up to 2 weeks.

Raspberry-Oat Streusel Bars

Maintaining a stable gastrointestinal tract is important to prevent symptoms of UC. These bars contain fiber from whole grains and berries, which feed beneficial gut bacteria and help maintain a healthy intestinal wall. These snack bars can be prepared in just 15 minutes. They are also delicious!

Serving Size: 16

Prep and Cook Time: 1 hr.

INGREDIENTS

- 2 cups fresh raspberries

- Cooking spray
- 3 Tbsp. pure maple syrup
- 2 Tbsp. corn starch
- 5 Tbsp unsalted butter, melted
- 1 ½ cups old-fashioned rolled oats
- 1 cup white whole-wheat flour
- 1 tsp. vanilla extract
- ¾ cup coconut sugar (or brown sugar)
- ¾ tsp. kosher salt
- 3 Tbsp. extra-virgin olive oil

Nutrition Information

Per serving: *164 Calories; 7g Fat; 2g Saturated Fat; 10mg Cholesterol; 91mg Sodium; 24g Carbohydrate; 3g Fiber; 2g Protein; 12g Sugar; 18mg Calcium; 1mg Iron; 63mg Potassium*

DIRECTIONS

STEP 1

Mix the maple syrup, raspberries, cornstarch and 3 tablespoons of water in a medium pot. Simmer and mash the berries to break them down. Reduce the heat to medium-low level; cook until thick, for about 5 minutes. Remove from the heat and let cool slightly.

STEP 2

Preheat the oven to 350°F. Coat an 11" x 7" baking pan with cooking spray. In a medium bowl, Mix the oats, salt, coconut sugar and flour. Add butter, oil and vanilla. Reserve a ⅔ cup of oatmeal mixture.

STEP 3

Sprinkle the remaining oat mixture evenly on the prepared plate; press firmly. Spread the raspberry mixture evenly on top, and then sprinkle the remaining oat mixture on the raspberries. Bake for about 35 minutes until it turns light brown.

STEP 4

Cool completely on the wire rack. Cut into 16 squares. Store in an airtight container for up to 3 days.

No-Bake Brownie Bites

If you are a fan of Nutella, you will love the chocolate hazelnut flavor in these energy snacks. When you have ulcerative colitis, limiting sugar supplementation is an important way to stop inflammation. These bites are naturally sweetened by dates and also increase the concentrated dose of fiber, vitamins and minerals.

Serving Size: 10

Prep and Cook Time: 15 min.

INGREDIENTS

- 12 pitted Medjool dates
- ½ cup raw cashews
- 2 Tbsp. cocoa powder
- ¼ cup almond butter
- ½ cup hazelnuts
- ½ tsp. vanilla extract
- ¼ tsp. kosher salt

Nutrition Information

Per serving: *183 Calories; 10g Fat; 1g Saturated Fat; 0mg Cholesterol; 70mg*
Sodium; 23g Carbohydrate; 4g Fiber; 4g Protein; 17g Sugar; 47mg Calcium; 1mg Iron; 214mg Potassium

DIRECTIONS

STEP 1

Put the dates, hazelnuts and cashews in a food processor; process until mixture is finely chopped. Add vanilla, almond butter, cocoa powder, and salt; process until mixture just starts to clump together.

STEP 2

Roll the mixture into 1 Tbsp. balls and chill until ready to serve. Store in an airtight container in the refrigerator for up to 14 days.

Cucumber and Tuna-Salad Sushi Rolls

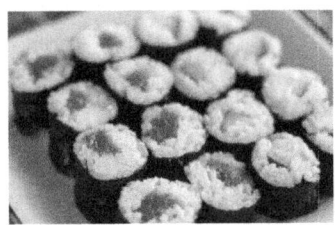 Use pop-up high-protein snacks between meals to keep you energized. When you need some fillings that will not cause harm, you can choose this snack. Cucumber has the lowest fiber content and high-water content, so it is easy to digest. During UC outbreaks, tuna will provide you with a healthy protein dose to make you satisfied.

Serving Size: 1

Prep and Cook Time: 15 min.

INGREDIENTS

- 1 (3-oz.) pouch wild albacore tuna, drained
- 2 tsp. mayonnaise
- ½ tsp. Dijon mustard
- ¼ tsp. kosher salt
- ¼ tsp. lemon zest, plus 1 tsp. fresh lemon juice
- ¼ tsp. black pepper
- 1 English cucumber, halved crosswise

Nutrition Information

Per serving: *200 Calories; 8g Fat; 1g Saturated Fat; 41mg Cholesterol; 874mg Sodium; 7g Carbohydrate; 3g Fiber; 30g Protein; 41g Sugar; 64mg Calcium; 1mg Iron; 418mg Potassium*

DIRECTIONS

STEP 1

Put the tuna, lemon zest, juice, mustard, salt, mayonnaise and pepper in bowl; mix well.

STEP 2

Trim off cucumber ends; reserve for another use. Slice cucumber halves lengthwise into 10 ⅛-inch-thick ribbons using any slicer. Place the slices flat on a cutting board.

STEP 3

Sprinkle 2 tsp. of the tuna mixture towards one end of each cucumber ribbon, about 1 inch from the edge. Wrap edge of each cucumber ribbon over tuna and continue to roll into sushi-sized bites.

Banana-Chia Pudding

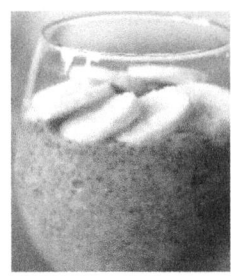 Chia seeds are one of the richest plant sources of ALA (a type of omega-3 fatty acid) and help fight inflammation caused by diseases such as ulcerative colitis. Adding bananas to the pudding can provide prebiotic fiber to promote intestinal health.

Serving Size: 2

Prep and Cook Time: 6 hr. 10 min.

INGREDIENTS

- 2 small ripe bananas, divided
- 1 Tbsp. pure maple syrup
- 4 Tbsp. chia seeds
- 1 Tbsp. unsweetened cocoa powder
- 4 Tbsp. chopped walnuts
- 1 cup unsweetened vanilla almond milk
- 2 Tbsp. cacao nibs

Nutrition Information

Per serving: 326 Calories; 7g Fat; 5g Saturated Fat; 0mg Cholesterol; 97mg

Sodium; 50g Carbohydrate; 15g Fiber; 9g Protein; 21g Sugar; 266mg Calcium; 4mg Iron; 620mg Potassium

DIRECTIONS

STEP 1

Put a banana in a bowl and mash it thoroughly with a fork. Transfer to a glass bottle, add Chia seeds, maple syrup, cocoa powder and almond milk. Close the lid and shake to combine. Let stand for 5 minutes, remove cover and stir with a spoon to break clumps. Cover and refrigerate overnight, or at least 6 hours.

STEP 2

Pour the chia pudding equally in two bowls. Cut the remaining bananas into thin slices and divide into the two bowls. Garnish each with 2 tablespoons of chopped walnuts and a tablespoon of cocoa nibs.

21-DAY COMPLETE DIET GUIDE \ MEAL PLAN FOR ULCERATIVE COLITIS AND CROHN'S

Week1

	SUNDAY
Breakfast (8:00-8:30AM)	Brown Bread and Egg Sandwich + an Apple
Mid-Meal (11:00-11:30AM)	Cherry Almond-Butter Bars with 1 Glass of Coconut Water
Lunch (2:00-2:30PM)	2 Roti with A Cup Of Soy Bean Curry + 1/2 Cup Curd
Evening (4:00-4:30PM)	A Cup of Tea + 1 Roasted Papad/ Murmure/ Bhuna Chana or Roasted Namkeen
Dinner (8:00-8:30PM)	2 Roti + Bottle Gourd Curry \ Red Curry Chicken and Rice
	MONDAY

Breakfast (8:00-8:30AM)	1 Brown Bread Potato Sandwich + 1 Cup Low-Fat Curd
Mid-Meal (11:00-11:30AM)	Oatmeal Pancake with 1 Cup of Chhach
Lunch (2:00-2:30PM)	Rice (1 Plate) + Fish/ Chicken Curry (1 Cup) + Cucumber Salad
Evening (4:00-4:30PM)	(1 cup) Tea + 1 Roasted Papad/ murmure/ bhunachana or roasted namkeen
Dinner (8:00-8:30PM)	2 Roti + Pointed Gourd Curry (a cup)/Chicken Piccata Pasta
TUESDAY	
Breakfast (8:00-8:30AM)	1 Brown bread vegetable sandwich + 1 pear
Mid-Meal (11:00-11:30AM)	1 Cup Chana sattu
Lunch (2:00-2:30PM)	2 Roti with Mushroom and 1 cup Green pea Curry + 1/2 cup curd

Evening (4:00-4:30PM)	Tea with 1 Roasted Papad/ murmure/ bhunachana or roasted namkeen
Dinner (8:00-8:30PM)	2 Roti with Beetroot Curry (1 Cup) \ Chil Shrimp Tacos

WEDNESDAY

Breakfast (8:00-8:30AM)	Vegetable Poha (1 plate) + a glass of Pomegranate juice
Mid-Meal (11:00-11:30AM)	1 cup Chhach
Lunch (2:00-2:30PM)	2 Roti and Chana Dal (a cup) plus 1 cup karela vegetable and green chutney
Evening (4:00-4:30PM)	Tea (a cup) with 1 Roasted Papad/ murmure/ bhunachana or roasted namkeen

Dinner (8:00-8:30PM)	2 Roti with Potato and Beans Curry (1 cup)
	THURSDAY

Breakfast (8:00-8:30AM)	1 Brown bread Toasted and Scrambled Egg + an apple
Mid-Meal (11:00-11:30AM)	2 biscuits with coconut water (a glass)
Lunch (2:00-2:30PM)	Rice (1 plate) with kidney beans Curry (1 cup) + green chutney
Evening (4:00-4:30PM)	Tea with 1 Roasted Papad/ murmure/ bhunachana or roasted namkeen
Dinner (8:00-8:30PM)	Roti (2) with lotus stem (1 cup) and green chutney
Friday	
Breakfast (8:00-8:30AM)	Mashed Potato n Carrot Sandwich with 1 cup curd
Mid-Meal (11:00 AM)	1 cup Chhach
Lunch (2:002:30PM)	Roti (2) with Moong Dal (1 cup) + 1 cup lady finger + green chutney

Evening (4:00-4:30PM)	Tea and 1 Roasted Papad/ murmure/ bhunachana or roasted namkeen
Dinner (8:00-8:30PM)	Roti and (1 cup) Potato n Drumstick Curry
Saturday	
Breakfast (8:00-8:30AM)	2 Besan Cheela with paneer stuffing with (1 glass) Pomegranate Juice
Mid-Meal (11:00-11:30AM)	1 cup Chana sattu
Lunch (2:00-2:30PM)	2 Roti with Chicken Curry (1 cup) and onion salad
Evening (4:00-4:30PM)	Tea (1 cup) + 1 Roasted Papad/ murmure/ bhunachana/ roasted namkeen
Dinner (8:00-8:30PM)	Roti (2) and Broad Beans Curry (1 cup)

Week2

	SUNDAY
Breakfast (8:008:30AM)	Whole-grain Morning glory muffins1 / Brown Bread Potato Sandwich + 1 Cup Low-Fat Curd
Mid-Meal (11:0011:30AM)	1 Cup of Chhach
Lunch (2:002:30PM)	Rice (1 Plate) + Fish/ Chicken Curry (1 Cup) + Cucumber Salad
Evening (4:004:30PM)	(1 cup) Tea + 1 Roasted Papad/ murmure/ bhunachana or roasted namkeen
Dinner (8:008:30PM)	2 Roti + Pointed Gourd Curry (a cup)
	MONDAY

Breakfast (8:00-8:30AM)	Brown Bread and Egg Sandwich + an Apple
Mid-Meal (11:00-11:30AM)	2 Biscuits + 1 Glass of Coconut Water
Lunch (2:00-2:30PM)	2 Roti with A Cup Of Soy Bean Curry + 1/2 Cup Curd
Evening (4:00-4:30PM)	A Cup of Tea + 1 Roasted Papad/ Murmure/ Bhuna Chana or Roasted Namkeen
Dinner (8:00-8:30PM)	2 Roti + Bottle Gourd Curry

TUESDAY

Breakfast (8:00-8:30AM)	1 Brown bread vegetable sandwich + 1 pear
Mid-Meal (11:00-11:30AM)	1 Cup Chana sattu
Lunch (2:00-2:30PM)	2 Roti with Mushroom and 1 cup Green pea Curry + 1/2 cup curd
Evening (4:00-4:30PM)	Tea with 1 Roasted Papad/ murmure/ bhuna chana or roasted namkeen
Dinner (8:00-8:30PM)	2 Roti with Beetroot Curry (1 cup)

WEDNESDAY

Breakfast (8:00o8:30AM)	Vegetable Poha (1 plate) + a glass of Pomegranate juice
Mid-Meal (11:00o11:30AM)	1 cup Chhach
Lunch (2:00o2:30PM)	2 Roti and Chana Dal (a cup) plus 1 cup karela vegetable and green chutney
Evening (4:00o4:30PM)	Tea (a cup) with 1 Roasted Papad/ murmure/ bhunachana or roasted namkeen
Dinner (8:00o8:30PM)	2 Roti with Potato and Beans Curry (1 cup)
THURSDAY	
Breakfast (8:00o8:30AM)	1 Brown bread Toasted and Scrambled Egg + an apple
Mid-Meal (11:00o11:30AM)	2 biscuits with coconut water (a glass)

Lunch (2:002:30PM)	Rice (1 plate) with kidney beans Curry (1 cup) + green chutney
Evening (4:004:30PM)	Tea with 1 Roasted Papad/ murmure/ bhunachana or roasted namkeen
Dinner (8:008:30PM)	Roti (2) with lotus stem (1 cup) and green chutney
Friday	
Breakfast (8:008:30AM)	Mashed Potato n Carrot Sandwich with 1 cup curd
Mid-Meal (11:0011:30AM)	1 cup Chhach
Lunch (2:002:30PM)	Roti (2) with Moong Dal (1 cup) + 1 cup lady finger + green chutney
Evening (4:004:30PM)	Tea and 1 Roasted Papad/ murmure/ bhunachana or roasted namkeen

Dinner (8:00 8:30PM)	Roti and (1 cup) Potato n Drumstick Curry
Saturday	
Breakfast (8:00 8:30AM)	2 BesanCheela with paneer stuffing with (1 glass) Pomegranate Juice
Mid-Meal (11:00 11:30AM)	1 cup Chana sattu
Lunch (2:00 2:30PM)	2 Roti with Chicken Curry (1 cup) and onion salad
Evening (4:00 4:30PM)	Tea (1 cup) + 1 Roasted Papad/ murmure/ bhunachana/ roasted namkeen
Dinner (8:00 8:30PM)	Roti (2) and Broad Beans Curry (1 cup)

Week3

Create a personalized meal plan for this week. Its best you select from the meals you have eaten which didn't cause any discomfort. Don't forget to write down any of the recipes which you have or will prepare during the day or week. It is best you repeat any of the week. You can swap any listed meal with your favorite which does not trigger flare. Always stay hydrate at all time!

SUNDAY	
Breakfast (8:008:30AM)	
Mid-Meal (11:0011:30AM)	
Lunch (2:002:30PM)	
Evening (4:004:30PM)	

Dinner (8:008:30PM)	
MONDAY	
Breakfast	

(8:00-
8:30AM)

Mid-Meal
(11:00-
11:30AM)

Lunch
(2:00-
2:30PM)

Evening
(4:00-
4:30PM)

Dinner
(8:00-
8:30PM)

TUESDAY

Breakfast
(8:00-
8:30AM)

Mid-Meal
(11:00-
11:30AM)

Lunch
(2:00-
2:30PM)

Evening
(4:00-
4:30PM)

Dinner
(8:00-
8:30PM)

WEDNESDAY

Breakfast (8:00–8:30AM)	
Mid-Meal (11:00–11:30AM)	
Lunch (2:00–2:30PM)	
Evening (4:00–4:30PM)	
Dinner (8:00–8:30PM)	
THURSDAY	
Breakfast (8:00–8:30AM)	
Mid-Meal (11:00–11:30AM)	

Lunch
(2:00 2:30PM)

Evening

 (4:00 4:30PM)

Dinner
(8:00 8:30PM)

Friday

Breakfast
(8:00 8:30AM)

Mid-Meal
(11:00 11:30AM)

Lunch
(2:00 2:30PM)

Evening
(4:00 4:30PM)

Dinner (8:008:30PM)	
Saturday	
Breakfast (8:008:30AM)	
Mid-Meal (11:0011:30AM)	
Lunch (2:002:30PM)	
Evening (4:004:30PM)	
Dinner (8:008:30PM)	

Made in the USA
Las Vegas, NV
02 April 2022

46742919R00059